Table Of Contents

Chapter 1: Understanding Arthritis and Its Impact   **2**

Chapter 2: The Benefits of Yoga for Arthritis   **14**

Chapter 3: Getting Started with Yoga   **24**

Chapter 4: Foundational Yoga Poses for Arthritis   **35**

Chapter 5: Building Your Yoga Routine   **46**

Chapter 6: Yoga Sequences for Pain Relief   **57**

Chapter 7: Mindfulness and Meditation Techniques   **68**

Chapter 8: Overcoming Challenges in Your Practice   **79**

Chapter 9: Testimonials and Success Stories   **90**

Chapter 10: Resources and Further Reading   **101**

Chapter 1: Understanding Arthritis and Its Impact

What is Arthritis?

Arthritis is a term that encompasses various conditions characterized by inflammation of the joints, which can lead to pain, stiffness, and decreased mobility. The most common types include osteoarthritis and rheumatoid arthritis. Osteoarthritis is often associated with wear and tear on the joints, typically developing as people age. In contrast, rheumatoid arthritis is an autoimmune condition where the body's immune system mistakenly attacks the synovial membrane, leading to inflammation and joint damage. Understanding the nature of arthritis is essential for developing effective strategies for management and relief.

The symptoms of arthritis can vary widely, ranging from mild discomfort to debilitating pain. Common signs include swelling, tenderness, and a decreased range of motion in the affected joints. These symptoms can significantly impact daily activities, affecting quality of life and mental well-being. Individuals may experience fatigue and emotional stress as a result of chronic pain and the limitations imposed by their condition. Recognizing these symptoms is crucial for early diagnosis and intervention, which can help slow the progression of the disease.

Arthritis is not solely a physical ailment; it also has psychological and social dimensions. The chronic pain associated with arthritis can lead to feelings of isolation and depression. Many people with arthritis find themselves limiting their activities due to fear of pain or exacerbation of their symptoms. This can create a cycle of inactivity that further exacerbates both physical and emotional challenges. Therefore, addressing the holistic aspects of arthritis management is essential for improving overall well-being.

Yoga has emerged as a powerful tool for individuals with arthritis and autoimmune diseases. The gentle movements and breathing techniques inherent in yoga can alleviate pain, improve flexibility, and enhance overall physical function. Specific poses can be adapted to accommodate varying levels of ability and pain, making yoga accessible to a wide range of individuals. Furthermore, the meditative aspects of yoga can help reduce stress and anxiety, which are often heightened in those living with chronic conditions.

Incorporating yoga into the daily routine can provide individuals with a sense of control over their condition. Regular practice fosters not only physical benefits but also emotional resilience. By learning to listen to their bodies and respect their limits, individuals can cultivate a more positive relationship with their arthritis. The combination of physical movement, mindfulness, and community support found in yoga can empower those affected by arthritis, offering them tools for pain relief that extend beyond conventional treatments.

Types of Arthritis

Arthritis encompasses a wide range of conditions characterized by inflammation and pain in the joints. The two most common types are osteoarthritis and rheumatoid arthritis, each with distinct causes, symptoms, and treatment approaches. Osteoarthritis is primarily a degenerative joint disease that occurs when the cartilage that cushions the joints wears down over time. This condition is often associated with aging and can result from repetitive stress on the joints. Symptoms typically include stiffness, swelling, and decreased range of motion, which can significantly impact daily activities and quality of life.

Rheumatoid arthritis, on the other hand, is an autoimmune disorder in which the immune system mistakenly attacks the body's own joint tissues. This condition can affect multiple joints simultaneously and often leads to systemic symptoms such as fatigue and fever. Unlike osteoarthritis, rheumatoid arthritis can occur at any age and may lead to significant joint damage if not properly managed. Treatment for rheumatoid arthritis often involves medications that control inflammation and suppress the immune response, highlighting the importance of early diagnosis and intervention.

Psoriatic arthritis is another type of arthritis that occurs in some individuals with psoriasis, a skin condition characterized by red, scaly patches. This form of arthritis can lead to joint inflammation as well as skin symptoms, and it may affect any part of the body, including the spine. The severity of psoriatic arthritis can vary greatly, with some individuals experiencing mild symptoms while others face debilitating pain and mobility issues. Treatment typically focuses on managing both skin and joint symptoms, emphasizing the need for a comprehensive approach to care.

Ankylosing spondylitis is a type of inflammatory arthritis that primarily affects the spine and the sacroiliac joints, which connect the spine to the pelvis. This condition is characterized by chronic pain and stiffness, particularly in the lower back, and can lead to a fusion of the vertebrae over time. Early detection and intervention are crucial, as lifestyle modifications, physical therapy, and specific exercises can help manage symptoms and improve mobility. Individuals with ankylosing spondylitis often benefit from incorporating yoga into their daily routines, as gentle stretching and strengthening can alleviate discomfort.

Gout is a type of arthritis that results from the accumulation of uric acid crystals in the joints, often leading to sudden and severe pain, redness, and swelling. It is commonly associated with dietary factors and can be triggered by certain foods, alcohol, or dehydration. Gout attacks can be extremely painful and may require medication to reduce inflammation and manage pain. Lifestyle changes, including dietary modifications and hydration, play a crucial role in preventing future flare-ups. Understanding the various types of arthritis is essential for those affected, as it enables individuals to explore appropriate treatment options, including the integration of yoga practices tailored to their specific condition.

Symptoms and Diagnosis

Arthritis encompasses a range of conditions that result in inflammation and pain in the joints, leading to various debilitating symptoms. The most common forms of arthritis include osteoarthritis and rheumatoid arthritis, each presenting unique characteristics. Individuals may experience symptoms such as joint pain, stiffness, swelling, and reduced range of motion. These symptoms can significantly impact daily activities and quality of life, making it essential for individuals to recognize the signs early on for effective management.

In addition to joint-related symptoms, individuals with arthritis may also experience systemic symptoms, particularly in autoimmune types like rheumatoid arthritis. These can include fatigue, fever, and malaise, which may not be directly related to joint issues but indicate an underlying inflammatory process. Recognizing these systemic symptoms can aid in distinguishing between different types of arthritis and in understanding the overall impact of the disease on the body.

Diagnosis of arthritis typically begins with a comprehensive medical history and physical examination. Healthcare professionals will often inquire about the onset, duration, and nature of symptoms, as well as any family history of autoimmune diseases. A thorough examination may reveal signs of swelling, tenderness, or deformity in affected joints. Based on initial findings, further diagnostic tests such as blood tests, imaging studies, or joint aspiration may be conducted to confirm the diagnosis and assess the extent of joint damage.

Blood tests are particularly vital in diagnosing autoimmune forms of arthritis. These tests may check for specific markers, such as rheumatoid factor or anti-citrullinated protein antibodies, which are often elevated in rheumatoid arthritis. Imaging studies such as X-rays, MRIs, or ultrasounds can help visualize joint damage and inflammation, providing crucial information for developing an effective treatment plan. The combination of clinical evaluation and laboratory results allows healthcare providers to differentiate between types of arthritis and tailor interventions accordingly.

Understanding the symptoms and the diagnostic process fosters a proactive approach to managing arthritis. For those integrating yoga into their treatment regimen, being aware of these aspects can enhance their practice by encouraging mindfulness and awareness of body signals. Yoga can serve as a complementary therapy, focusing on gentle movements and breathwork to alleviate pain and improve joint function. By recognizing symptoms early and seeking appropriate diagnosis, individuals can better navigate their journey with arthritis and explore therapeutic options, including yoga, that support their overall well-being.

The Connection Between Arthritis and Autoimmune Diseases

Arthritis and autoimmune diseases share a complex and often intertwined relationship that has significant implications for those affected by these conditions. At its core, arthritis is characterized by inflammation of the joints, leading to pain and stiffness. Autoimmune diseases occur when the immune system mistakenly attacks the body's own tissues. Many forms of arthritis, such as rheumatoid arthritis and psoriatic arthritis, are classified as autoimmune diseases, highlighting a critical connection between the two. Understanding this relationship is essential for developing effective management strategies, including the incorporation of yoga as a complementary therapy.

The immune system plays a pivotal role in the inflammation associated with arthritis. In autoimmune forms of arthritis, the immune system's dysregulation leads to the production of antibodies that target joint tissues. This results in chronic inflammation, which can cause significant joint damage over time if not properly managed.

Patients with autoimmune arthritis often experience flare-ups, where symptoms worsen unpredictably. Recognizing the autoimmune component can guide treatment approaches, emphasizing the need for both medical interventions and lifestyle changes, such as yoga, to help mitigate these symptoms.

Yoga offers a holistic approach to managing arthritis and autoimmune diseases by promoting both physical and mental well-being. The gentle movements and stretches involved in yoga can enhance flexibility, strengthen muscles around the joints, and improve overall mobility. Furthermore, practices such as mindful breathing and meditation can reduce stress, which is known to exacerbate inflammation. This dual benefit of physical and mental relief makes yoga an ideal practice for individuals suffering from the challenges posed by arthritis and autoimmune conditions.

Research indicates that regular engagement in yoga can lead to significant improvements in pain levels, joint function, and quality of life for those with arthritis. Studies have shown that participants who practiced yoga experienced reduced levels of inflammatory markers in their bodies, suggesting a physiological benefit that extends beyond mere pain relief.

Additionally, the social aspect of participating in group yoga classes can foster a sense of community and support, which is invaluable for individuals managing chronic conditions. This connection can alleviate feelings of isolation that often accompany chronic illnesses.

Incorporating yoga into the management plan for arthritis and autoimmune diseases can empower individuals to take an active role in their health. It encourages a proactive approach to wellness, combining physical activity with stress management techniques. By understanding the connection between arthritis and autoimmune diseases, individuals can better appreciate the importance of holistic practices like yoga, which not only address physical symptoms but also promote emotional resilience. As research continues to illuminate these connections, the integration of yoga into arthritis management will likely become an increasingly recognized and valuable resource for those seeking relief and improved quality of life.

Chapter 2: The Benefits of Yoga for Arthritis

How Yoga Can Help Manage Pain

Yoga can be an effective complementary approach to managing pain associated with arthritis and autoimmune diseases. Through a combination of gentle movement, focused breathing, and mindfulness, yoga helps to alleviate discomfort, improve flexibility, and enhance overall well-being. The practice encourages a deeper connection between the mind and body, which can be particularly beneficial in coping with the chronic pain often experienced by individuals with these conditions.

One of the primary mechanisms by which yoga aids in pain management is through the promotion of relaxation and stress reduction. Chronic pain can frequently be exacerbated by stress and anxiety, creating a vicious cycle that can be difficult to break. Yoga techniques such as deep breathing and meditation activate the parasympathetic nervous system, which calms the body and reduces the perception of pain. This shift in focus from pain to relaxation can empower individuals to manage their symptoms more effectively.

Moreover, yoga enhances physical mobility, which is crucial for those with arthritis and related conditions. Many yoga poses are designed to increase joint range of motion and build strength without placing excessive strain on the body. By practicing these poses regularly, individuals can experience improved flexibility, which may help alleviate stiffness and discomfort in affected joints. This increased mobility can lead to a more active lifestyle, further contributing to pain relief and overall health.

In addition to physical benefits, yoga fosters a sense of community and support. Participating in group classes or online sessions can help individuals feel less isolated in their struggles with chronic pain. Sharing experiences with others who face similar challenges creates a supportive environment that encourages resilience and hope. The camaraderie found in yoga classes can be a vital source of motivation, helping individuals to stay committed to their practice and pain management strategies.

Finally, integrating yoga into a daily routine can promote a greater awareness of one's body and its signals. This mindfulness allows individuals to recognize patterns in their pain and understand how certain activities or stressors may contribute to flare-ups. By cultivating this awareness, practitioners can make informed choices about their movements and lifestyle, leading to improved self-management of pain. Overall, yoga serves as a holistic approach to managing pain, offering physical, emotional, and social benefits that can significantly enhance the quality of life for those living with arthritis and autoimmune diseases.

Improving Flexibility and Strength

Improving flexibility and strength is essential for individuals with arthritis and autoimmune diseases, as it can significantly enhance overall functionality and quality of life. Yoga, with its gentle movements and focus on breath control, provides a holistic approach to addressing these needs. By incorporating specific poses into a regular practice, individuals can work towards increased range of motion and muscular strength, which can alleviate some of the discomfort associated with their conditions.

Flexibility is crucial in managing arthritis symptoms. Stiffness in joints can often lead to decreased mobility, making everyday activities challenging. Yoga poses such as cat-cow, child's pose, and gentle forward bends can help stretch the muscles surrounding the joints, promoting greater elasticity. Practicing these poses consistently enables individuals to experience less tightness and increased joint mobility, contributing to better overall movement patterns.

Strength is equally important for those with arthritis or autoimmune diseases. Building strength in the muscles that support the joints can reduce the strain placed on them. Poses like warrior II, chair pose, and bridge pose are effective in strengthening the legs, core, and back. By focusing on these muscle groups, individuals can develop a stabilizing foundation that helps protect the joints from excessive wear and tear. Moreover, enhanced strength can lead to improved balance, reducing the risk of falls and injuries.

In addition to physical benefits, the mental aspect of yoga cannot be overlooked. The practice encourages mindfulness and body awareness, which can foster a more positive relationship with one's body. Individuals often learn to listen to their bodies and recognize their limits, allowing for a more adaptive approach to their yoga practice. This mental shift can result in increased confidence and motivation to engage in physical activity, further supporting flexibility and strength development.

Ultimately, improving flexibility and strength through yoga is a gradual process that requires patience and consistency. Individuals with arthritis and autoimmune diseases should approach their practice with a sense of ease, prioritizing gentle movements and modifications as needed. By integrating these principles into their routine, they can cultivate a more resilient body, reduce pain levels, and enhance their overall well-being, making yoga an invaluable component of their self-care regimen.

Stress Reduction Through Mindfulness

Mindfulness is a powerful tool that can significantly reduce stress, particularly for individuals coping with arthritis and autoimmune diseases. Stress often exacerbates physical symptoms and can lead to a cycle of pain and emotional turmoil. By incorporating mindfulness practices into daily routines, individuals can cultivate a greater sense of awareness and control over their bodies and minds. This approach allows for the acknowledgment of discomfort without judgment, creating a space for healing and acceptance.

At its core, mindfulness involves being present in the moment, which can be particularly beneficial for those dealing with chronic pain. Practicing mindfulness encourages individuals to focus on their breath and bodily sensations while observing thoughts and feelings without becoming overwhelmed by them. This practice can help reduce anxiety and promote relaxation, which are crucial for managing the symptoms associated with arthritis and autoimmune disorders. Simple techniques such as guided meditations or mindful breathing exercises can be integrated into yoga sessions, enhancing both mental and physical well-being.

Incorporating mindfulness into yoga practice can also deepen the connection between mind and body. For individuals with arthritis, gentle yoga poses combined with mindful attention can help improve flexibility and strength while simultaneously fostering a sense of inner peace. The focus on breath during yoga encourages practitioners to stay engaged with their bodies, allowing them to listen to what feels good and what doesn't. This awareness is essential for preventing injury and promoting a positive yoga experience, leading to a more sustainable practice.

Moreover, mindfulness can serve as a valuable tool for emotional regulation. Chronic illness often brings about feelings of frustration, sadness, and isolation. Mindfulness teaches individuals to acknowledge these emotions without suppressing them, fostering a healthier relationship with their feelings. By cultivating self-compassion and acceptance, practitioners can reduce the emotional burden of living with arthritis or an autoimmune disease, ultimately contributing to a more balanced and fulfilling life.

Finally, the benefits of mindfulness extend beyond the yoga mat. By integrating mindfulness practices into everyday activities, individuals can enhance their overall quality of life. Simple actions such as mindful eating, walking, or even engaging in conversations can transform mundane experiences into opportunities for mindfulness. Over time, these practices can lead to a more resilient mindset, better coping strategies, and a significant reduction in stress, making them invaluable for anyone managing the challenges of arthritis and autoimmune diseases.

Enhancing Overall Well-Being

Enhancing overall well-being is a holistic approach that integrates physical, mental, and emotional health, particularly for individuals coping with arthritis and autoimmune diseases. The practice of yoga offers a unique avenue to foster this well-being, combining gentle movements, breath control, and mindfulness. Each of these elements plays a crucial role in alleviating the physical discomfort associated with arthritis while simultaneously promoting a sense of peace and balance in daily life.

Physical activity is essential for managing arthritis, and yoga provides a low-impact option that can be tailored to individual needs. Certain poses can improve flexibility, strength, and balance, which are vital for maintaining joint function and reducing stiffness. For example, poses such as Cat-Cow and Child's Pose allow for gentle stretching of the spine and surrounding muscles, enhancing mobility without placing undue stress on the joints. Practicing these movements regularly can help to maintain a range of motion and potentially reduce the frequency of flare-ups associated with inflammatory conditions.

In addition to physical benefits, the breathwork involved in yoga practice is particularly beneficial for those managing chronic pain. Techniques such as diaphragmatic breathing or alternate nostril breathing can activate the body's relaxation response, reducing stress and anxiety levels. This is important because stress can exacerbate symptoms of arthritis and other autoimmune diseases. By incorporating breath control into their routine, practitioners can cultivate a sense of calm and improve their overall emotional resilience, making it easier to cope with the challenges of living with chronic illness.

Mindfulness is another key aspect of yoga that greatly contributes to enhancing overall well-being. Engaging in mindful movement encourages individuals to be present in their bodies and aware of their sensations, fostering a deeper connection to their physical selves. This practice can help shift focus away from pain and discomfort, allowing for a more positive outlook on one's condition. Meditation and mindfulness techniques can also assist in managing negative thought patterns, leading to improved mental health and a greater sense of empowerment over one's health journey.

Lastly, the community aspect of yoga can provide essential social support for those dealing with arthritis and autoimmune diseases. Participating in group classes or workshops fosters connections with others who share similar experiences, creating a sense of belonging and understanding. This social interaction can be invaluable in combating feelings of isolation that often accompany chronic illness. By enhancing overall well-being through yoga, individuals not only address their physical symptoms but also nurture their mental and emotional health, creating a comprehensive framework for living well despite challenges.

Chapter 3: Getting Started with Yoga

Preparing for Your Yoga Practice

Preparing for your yoga practice is essential, especially for individuals managing arthritis and autoimmune diseases. The right preparation can enhance your experience, making it more beneficial and enjoyable. Start by creating a dedicated space for your practice. This space should be quiet, free from distractions, and equipped with the necessary tools such as a yoga mat, blocks, and straps. Ensure the area is well-lit, but not too bright, to promote a calming atmosphere. Consider adding supportive elements like cushions or blankets to enhance comfort during your practice.

Before you begin, it is vital to check in with your body. Take a moment to assess how you feel physically and mentally. Understanding your current state can help you modify poses according to your comfort level. If you are experiencing increased pain or fatigue, listen to your body and adjust your practice accordingly. A gentle approach is particularly important for those with arthritis, as it allows for a more mindful and responsive practice that respects your body's limits.

Warm-up exercises can significantly benefit your yoga session. Gentle movements, such as neck rolls, shoulder shrugs, and wrist rotations, can help prepare your joints and muscles. These warm-ups increase blood flow and flexibility, reducing the risk of injury and enhancing your overall range of motion. Engaging in deep, mindful breathing during this time can further center your mind and body, setting a positive tone for the rest of your practice.

Incorporating modifications and props into your yoga routine is a crucial aspect of preparing for your practice. Props such as blocks can provide support in various poses, allowing you to maintain proper alignment without straining your body. It's essential to remember that yoga is not about perfection; it is about finding what works best for you. Experiment with different modifications until you discover the most comfortable and effective options for your body.

Finally, establishing a routine can help reinforce your commitment to your yoga practice. Aim to practice regularly, even if it is for a short duration. Consistency can lead to improved flexibility, strength, and overall well-being. Additionally, consider integrating mindfulness techniques into your routine, such as meditation or guided imagery, to enhance your mental focus and relaxation. By preparing effectively for your yoga practice, you can create a nurturing environment that supports your journey towards pain relief and improved quality of life.

Choosing the Right Space

Choosing the right space for practicing yoga is crucial for individuals living with arthritis and autoimmune diseases. A well-considered environment can significantly enhance the experience and effectiveness of each session. Factors such as accessibility, comfort, and ambiance play pivotal roles in ensuring that the practice is both enjoyable and beneficial. It is essential to create a space that accommodates specific physical needs while promoting relaxation and focus.

Accessibility is the foremost consideration when selecting a practice space. Individuals with arthritis may have limitations in mobility, which makes it important to choose an area that is easily reachable without excessive strain. Ideally, the space should be free from obstacles, ensuring that individuals can move around safely and confidently. Whether practicing at home or in a communal setting, having a clear path and avoiding clutter will help to prevent falls and injuries, which are significant concerns for those with joint issues.

Comfort is another vital aspect of the chosen space. This includes not only physical comfort but also emotional comfort. The surface on which one practices should provide adequate support; a yoga mat that is cushioned yet stable can help alleviate pressure on joints. Additionally, ensuring that the temperature of the room is conducive to relaxation can enhance the overall experience. A space that is too hot or too cold may distract from the practice and deter individuals from engaging fully.

Ambiance also contributes significantly to the effectiveness of yoga practice. A calming environment can help reduce stress, which is particularly important for individuals with autoimmune diseases, as stress can exacerbate symptoms. Soft lighting, soothing colors, and minimal noise can create a serene atmosphere. Incorporating elements such as plants or calming scents can further enhance the environment, making it inviting and conducive to mindfulness and relaxation.

Finally, personalization of the space can foster a deeper connection to the practice. Adding personal touches such as photographs, inspiring quotes, or meaningful objects can create a sense of ownership and encourage regular practice. Additionally, having necessary props within reach—such as blocks, straps, or cushions—can facilitate ease of movement and adaptation of poses, making yoga more accessible and effective for those managing arthritis and autoimmune conditions. By thoughtfully selecting and personalizing the space, practitioners can create an environment that supports their well-being and enhances their yoga journey.

Essential Equipment and Props

When embarking on a yoga journey specifically tailored for individuals with arthritis and autoimmune diseases, having the right equipment and props can significantly enhance the practice. Essential tools can provide support, improve accessibility, and facilitate deeper relaxation. First and foremost, a good quality yoga mat is crucial. It offers a non-slip surface that ensures stability during poses, reducing the risk of falls and injuries. A mat with adequate cushioning is beneficial for those with joint pain, as it provides additional comfort for sensitive knees and wrists.

Yoga blocks are another invaluable resource for practitioners with limited flexibility or strength. These props can be used to modify poses, bringing the ground closer and allowing for a more comfortable alignment. By placing a block under the hands in forward bends or under the hips in seated poses, individuals can perform movements without straining their joints. Blocks can also be stacked to create a higher surface, making transitions smoother and reducing the effort required to reach the floor.

Straps are equally important in a yoga toolkit. These versatile aids assist in maintaining proper alignment and extending reach during poses. For instance, a strap can be looped around the foot in seated stretches, allowing for greater extension without excessive strain on the joints. This is particularly beneficial for those who may struggle with tight muscles or limited range of motion. Using straps encourages individuals to explore their flexibility safely, promoting gradual improvements over time.

Additionally, cushions and bolsters play a vital role in restorative practices and relaxation techniques. These props provide support in seated and reclining positions, enabling practitioners to maintain comfort while holding poses for extended periods. A bolster can be placed under the knees in a supine position to relieve pressure on the lower back or used to elevate the hips in seated poses to promote better posture. This enhanced support helps create a nurturing environment conducive to healing and stress relief.

Finally, blankets can be easily incorporated into a yoga routine for added warmth and comfort. They can be used to pad joints, providing a softer surface during seated or kneeling poses. Blankets can also serve as props for restorative poses, offering gentle support and promoting relaxation. By creating a comfortable and supportive practice space with the right equipment, individuals with arthritis and autoimmune diseases can engage in yoga with confidence, ultimately leading to improved mobility and pain relief.

Safety Guidelines for Practicing Yoga

Safety is paramount when practicing yoga, especially for individuals with arthritis and autoimmune diseases. The unique challenges posed by these conditions necessitate a mindful approach to yoga, ensuring that each pose is performed safely and effectively. It is essential to listen to your body and recognize its limitations. This awareness can help prevent injuries and make the practice more enjoyable and beneficial. Always prioritize comfort over striving for perfection in each pose, and be willing to modify or skip poses that cause discomfort.

Before starting a yoga session, it is critical to consult with your healthcare provider or a qualified yoga instructor familiar with your medical history. They can provide insights into which poses are most suitable for your specific condition and how to adjust them to accommodate any limitations. This step is particularly important for individuals with severe symptoms or those who are new to yoga. A well-informed instructor can also guide you on proper alignment and techniques to avoid strain, promoting a safer practice.

Warm-up exercises are an essential component of any yoga routine, particularly for those with arthritis or autoimmune conditions. Gentle movements that increase blood flow to the joints can help prepare the body for deeper stretches and poses. Incorporating a few minutes of warm-up can enhance flexibility and reduce stiffness, making it easier to transition into more challenging positions. Additionally, using props such as blocks, straps, or cushions can provide support and stability, allowing for a more accessible practice.

During your yoga session, pay close attention to your breathing and body signals. Each inhale and exhale can help you maintain focus and calmness, which is crucial for managing pain. If you experience sharp pain or discomfort, it's important to stop immediately and reassess your position. Modifications can be made to reduce strain, such as using a chair for balance or performing poses seated instead of standing. Remember that yoga is not about achieving a specific stance; rather, it is about finding a practice that feels good for your body.

Finally, consider the environment in which you practice yoga. A calm and quiet space can contribute positively to your overall experience. Ensure that the area is free from distractions and that you have ample room to move without risk of injury. Practicing on a non-slip surface can also enhance stability and safety. By creating a supportive environment and adhering to these safety guidelines, you can enjoy the myriad benefits of yoga while effectively managing arthritis and autoimmune disease symptoms.

Chapter 4: Foundational Yoga Poses for Arthritis

Gentle Seated Poses

Gentle seated poses serve as an essential component of a yoga practice tailored for those living with arthritis and autoimmune diseases. These poses are designed to provide comfort while promoting flexibility, strength, and relaxation. By integrating gentle seated stretches into a daily routine, individuals can effectively manage pain and stiffness often associated with these conditions. The accessibility of seated poses allows practitioners to benefit from yoga's therapeutic effects without the strain that more demanding positions may impose.

One of the primary advantages of gentle seated poses is their ability to enhance joint mobility. Many seated poses focus on the major joints, including the hips, knees, and shoulders, allowing for a safe range of motion. For instance, seated forward bends can help stretch the spine and hamstrings while promoting increased blood circulation. This gentle movement can alleviate tension and stiffness in the body, providing relief to sensitive areas. Through consistent practice, individuals may find improved flexibility, which can contribute to a greater sense of ease in daily activities.

Moreover, gentle seated poses emphasize mindfulness and relaxation, which are particularly beneficial for those managing chronic pain. The act of focusing on breath and body awareness during these poses can help to reduce stress and anxiety, common companions of arthritis and autoimmune diseases. Techniques such as deep breathing and visualization can be incorporated into the practice, allowing individuals to cultivate a sense of peace and connection to their bodies. This mindful approach not only enhances physical well-being but also contributes to emotional resilience.

In addition to physical and mental benefits, gentle seated poses can also foster a sense of community and support when practiced in a group setting. Participating in yoga classes designed for individuals with arthritis creates an environment where practitioners can share experiences and encouragement. This communal aspect of yoga can play a vital role in combating the isolation that often accompanies chronic illness. Engaging with others in a safe space can lead to valuable connections, providing motivation and inspiration to maintain a regular practice.

Finally, it is essential to approach gentle seated poses with an understanding of personal limits and individual needs. Each person's experience with arthritis and autoimmune diseases is unique, and modifications may be necessary to ensure comfort and safety. Using props such as cushions or blankets can enhance stability and support during seated poses. Listening to the body and respecting its signals is paramount; if a pose causes discomfort, it may be beneficial to adjust or substitute it with a more suitable alternative. By fostering a compassionate and attentive practice, individuals can truly reap the rewards of yoga, finding relief and empowerment in their journey toward greater well-being.

Standing Poses for Stability

Standing poses play a crucial role in building stability and strength, particularly for individuals managing arthritis and autoimmune diseases. These poses can enhance balance, improve circulation, and foster a sense of grounding. When practiced mindfully, standing poses can help alleviate stiffness and discomfort while promoting overall joint health. It is essential for practitioners to listen to their bodies and modify poses as needed to ensure a safe and beneficial experience.

One of the most accessible standing poses is Tadasana, or Mountain Pose. This foundational pose encourages proper alignment and awareness of body mechanics. By standing tall with feet hip-width apart, grounding through the feet, and lengthening the spine, individuals can cultivate a sense of stability. Engaging the legs and core helps to distribute weight evenly, while the arms can rest gently by the sides or be lifted overhead. Tadasana serves as an excellent warm-up for other standing poses and can be practiced anytime for a quick energy boost.

Another beneficial standing pose is Virabhadrasana II, or Warrior II. This pose strengthens the legs and opens the hips, which can be particularly helpful for those experiencing joint stiffness. To enter Warrior II, practitioners should step one foot back, bend the front knee while keeping the back leg straight, and extend the arms parallel to the ground. The gaze can be directed over the front fingertips, promoting focus and concentration. This pose not only builds physical strength but also instills a sense of empowerment, making it a valuable addition to any yoga practice.

Tree Pose, or Vrikshasana, is an excellent option for enhancing balance and stability. This pose encourages practitioners to engage their core and focus on their breath while standing on one leg. By placing the opposite foot on the inner thigh or calf (avoiding the knee), individuals can work on their balance without straining their joints. The arms can be brought into a prayer position or lifted overhead for added challenge. Tree Pose invites a sense of calm and concentration, which can be particularly beneficial for those managing chronic pain or discomfort.

Incorporating standing poses into a regular yoga routine can significantly improve stability and overall well-being for individuals with arthritis and autoimmune diseases. As practitioners become more familiar with these poses, they can experiment with variations and modifications to suit their needs. It is essential to prioritize safety and comfort, allowing the body to adapt gradually to the demands of each pose. By cultivating a dedicated practice of standing poses, individuals can experience enhanced physical strength, improved balance, and a greater sense of connection to their bodies.

Restorative Poses for Relaxation

Restorative yoga poses offer a unique approach to relaxation that can be particularly beneficial for individuals with arthritis and autoimmune diseases. These poses emphasize gentle stretching and deep relaxation, allowing the body to release tension and promote healing. The key to restorative yoga is the use of props, such as blankets, bolsters, and blocks, which provide support and comfort, enabling practitioners to hold poses for an extended period. This sustained relaxation can help alleviate pain, reduce stress, and improve overall well-being.

One of the most effective restorative poses is supported child's pose. In this pose, practitioners kneel and sit back on their heels while resting their torso on a bolster or stack of blankets. This position encourages gentle stretching of the spine and hips while providing a calming effect on the nervous system. For individuals with arthritis, the support from props allows them to experience the benefits of the pose without straining their joints. Holding this pose for several minutes can create a deep sense of relaxation, fostering a connection between breath and body.

Another beneficial restorative pose is legs-up-the-wall pose. This pose involves lying on the floor with the legs extended vertically against a wall. This gentle inversion helps to reduce swelling in the legs and feet, which is a common concern for those with arthritis. Additionally, it promotes circulation and encourages lymphatic drainage. The restorative aspect of this pose is heightened when practitioners use a bolster under their lower back for added support, allowing them to relax deeply while enjoying the benefits of gravity.

Supported bridge pose is also an excellent choice for promoting relaxation and relieving tension in the lower back and hips. By placing a block or bolster under the sacrum, practitioners can gently lift their hips while keeping the spine in a neutral position. This pose encourages gentle stretching of the chest and shoulders, which can help counteract the tension that often builds in these areas due to pain or limited mobility. Maintaining this pose for several breaths can provide a profound sense of release and comfort, making it an ideal addition to a restorative yoga practice.

Incorporating restorative poses into a regular yoga routine can significantly benefit individuals managing arthritis and autoimmune diseases. These poses not only promote physical relief but also cultivate mental tranquility. Practicing restorative yoga encourages mindfulness and awareness of the body, helping individuals develop a greater understanding of their limitations while fostering a sense of empowerment. By prioritizing relaxation through these gentle poses, practitioners can create a nurturing environment for healing and self-care, essential for managing chronic conditions.

Modified Poses for Different Abilities

Yoga is a versatile practice that can be adapted to accommodate various abilities, especially for individuals living with arthritis and autoimmune diseases. The goal of modifying poses is to provide a safe and effective way to engage in yoga while minimizing discomfort and maximizing benefits. Understanding how to adjust traditional poses can help practitioners maintain their practice and improve their overall well-being.

One of the fundamental modifications involves using props such as blocks, straps, or bolsters. These tools can provide support and stability, making it easier to achieve and hold poses. For example, when practicing Downward Facing Dog, someone with limited wrist flexibility could place their hands on blocks to elevate them, reducing strain on the wrists while still allowing for the benefits of the pose. Similarly, using a chair for poses like Warrior I can provide a stable base for individuals who may struggle with balance or endurance.

Seated poses are particularly beneficial for those with joint pain or fatigue. Modifying standing poses into seated versions can help individuals participate in the practice without overexerting themselves. Poses like Seated Forward Bend or Seated Twist can be gentle alternatives that promote flexibility and relaxation without putting undue pressure on the joints. Additionally, focusing on breathwork and gentle movements while seated can enhance relaxation and reduce stress, which is crucial for managing the symptoms of arthritis and autoimmune conditions.

Gentle restorative poses also play a vital role in a modified yoga practice. Poses such as Supported Child's Pose or Legs-Up-the-Wall can be incredibly soothing and restorative. These poses can help alleviate tension and promote circulation without placing excessive strain on the body. Incorporating restorative practices into a regular routine can significantly enhance overall comfort and provide relief from pain and stiffness often associated with arthritis.

Finally, it is essential to encourage mindfulness and body awareness throughout the practice. Listening to one's body and making adjustments as needed is crucial for anyone with arthritis or autoimmune diseases. Practitioners should feel empowered to skip poses or modify them further based on their comfort levels. This approach not only fosters a safe environment but also nurtures a deeper connection with one's body, ultimately leading to a more fulfilling yoga experience tailored to individual needs.

Chapter 5: Building Your Yoga Routine

Creating a Balanced Practice

Creating a balanced yoga practice is essential for individuals living with arthritis and autoimmune diseases. A balanced practice not only alleviates pain but also promotes overall well-being. It's important to tailor your routine to address the unique challenges these conditions present. This involves incorporating a variety of poses that enhance flexibility, strength, and relaxation while being mindful of any limitations. Understanding your body's needs and responses is the first step in developing a sustainable practice that prioritizes both safety and effectiveness.

Incorporating restorative poses can significantly benefit those with arthritis and autoimmune diseases. These gentle poses, which focus on deep relaxation and mindful breathing, help reduce stress and inflammation in the body. Poses such as Child's Pose, Supported Bridge, and Legs-Up-the-Wall provide opportunities for the body to recharge and heal. These restorative practices are particularly valuable for individuals experiencing fatigue or flare-ups, as they allow for a connection to the breath and body without overstressing the joints.

Strength training is another crucial component of a balanced yoga practice. Building muscle strength around affected joints can lead to improved stability and reduced pain. Poses like Warrior I, Warrior II, and Chair Pose emphasize strength building while promoting proper alignment. It's important to approach these poses with caution, ensuring that the body is adequately warmed up and that modifications are used when necessary. This enables individuals to engage in strength training without risking injury or exacerbating their condition.

Flexibility is also an important aspect of a well-rounded practice. Gentle stretching can enhance range of motion and reduce stiffness associated with arthritis. Incorporating poses such as Cat-Cow, Seated Forward Bend, and Side Stretch encourages gentle elongation of the muscles and joints. Practitioners should listen to their bodies and avoid pushing into painful ranges of motion. Utilizing props like straps or blocks can aid in achieving poses without strain, making yoga more accessible and enjoyable.

Finally, a balanced practice should always include time for mindfulness and meditation. The mental aspect of managing arthritis and autoimmune diseases is often overlooked but is equally important. Techniques such as guided imagery, body scans, or simple breath awareness can provide significant relief from the mental burden of chronic pain. Establishing a calm and focused mindset enhances the overall experience of yoga, allowing individuals to cultivate resilience and a deeper connection to their bodies. By integrating these elements into a cohesive practice, individuals can create a holistic routine that supports their physical and emotional health.

Setting Realistic Goals

Setting realistic goals is essential for anyone managing arthritis and autoimmune diseases, especially when incorporating yoga into their daily routine. When starting a new practice, it is important to acknowledge individual limitations and understand that progress may be gradual. This approach not only fosters a positive mindset but also helps prevent frustration and potential injury. Setting attainable goals allows individuals to build confidence and maintain motivation, which are crucial elements for long-term success.

To begin setting realistic goals, individuals should first assess their current physical capabilities and limitations. This assessment can be done through self-reflection or by consulting with a healthcare professional. Understanding one's range of motion, pain levels, and overall physical condition will provide a clearer picture of what can be achieved through yoga practice. It's important to remember that everyone's journey is unique; thus, personalizing goals according to individual circumstances will lead to more meaningful accomplishments.

Once individuals have a clear understanding of their starting point, they can develop specific, measurable, achievable, relevant, and time-bound (SMART) goals. For instance, rather than aiming to master a challenging pose like Downward Dog within a week, an individual might set a goal to practice gentle stretches for ten minutes daily. This objective is not only realistic but also allows for gradual improvement. Celebrating small victories, such as increased flexibility or reduced pain levels, can significantly boost motivation and commitment to the practice.

Incorporating yoga into a daily routine should also consider external factors that may influence goal attainment. These factors include the time available for practice, the presence of support systems, and the overall environment. Setting goals that align with one's lifestyle will enhance the likelihood of consistency. For example, an individual might aim to join a local yoga class once a week or practice at home using guided videos that cater to their specific needs. Flexibility in goal setting can accommodate unexpected challenges, such as flare-ups or fatigue, ensuring that commitment to yoga remains manageable.

Lastly, it is important to revisit and adjust goals as necessary. As practitioners progress, their abilities and circumstances may change, necessitating a reevaluation of their aims. Regularly reflecting on and updating goals can help maintain motivation and ensure that the practice stays relevant to the individual's current needs. By fostering a realistic and adaptable approach to goal setting, individuals with arthritis and autoimmune diseases can harness the benefits of yoga, leading to improved pain relief and overall well-being.

Incorporating Breathwork and Meditation

Incorporating breathwork and meditation into your yoga practice can significantly enhance your experience, particularly for those managing arthritis and autoimmune diseases. Breathwork, or pranayama, focuses on the breath as a tool for enhancing physical and mental well-being. This technique not only helps to calm the nervous system but also encourages the body to relax and release tension. For individuals dealing with chronic pain, the ability to control one's breath can create a sense of empowerment and alleviate discomfort during yoga poses.

Meditation complements breathwork by fostering mindfulness and a deeper connection with the body. For those experiencing arthritis, mindfulness can be a powerful tool in recognizing pain signals without judgment. By honing in on the present moment, individuals can develop a greater awareness of their bodies, allowing them to modify movements and poses to suit their current state. This practice can reduce anxiety related to pain and help create a more positive mindset, which is essential for managing chronic conditions.

In the context of yoga, integrating breathwork and meditation can provide a holistic approach to pain management. Each yoga session can begin with focused breathing exercises, setting the tone for the practice ahead. This can include simple techniques such as diaphragmatic breathing or alternate nostril breathing, both of which promote relaxation and prepare the body for movement. Following these exercises with a short meditation session allows practitioners to center their thoughts and intentions, ensuring they are mentally prepared to engage in the physical aspects of yoga.

As you incorporate these practices into your routine, consider establishing a consistent schedule. Regular breathwork and meditation can enhance the benefits of your yoga poses, leading to improved flexibility, reduced stiffness, and a greater sense of overall well-being. Additionally, creating a dedicated space for these practices can enhance your focus and commitment. Whether it's a corner of your living room or a quiet outdoor space, having a designated area can help reinforce the importance of these practices in your daily life.

Finally, it is crucial to listen to your body during both breathwork and meditation. Individuals with arthritis and autoimmune diseases may experience fluctuations in their condition, making it essential to adapt practices accordingly. Allow yourself the flexibility to skip certain breaths or modify meditation techniques as needed. By honoring your body's signals and adjusting your practice, you can cultivate a supportive environment that promotes healing and comfort, ultimately enhancing your overall yoga experience.

Adapting Your Routine to Your Needs

Creating a yoga routine that adapts to your individual needs is essential for managing arthritis and autoimmune diseases. Each person's experience with these conditions varies, which means that a one-size-fits-all approach is rarely effective. By understanding your body, its limitations, and your personal goals, you can develop a practice that not only helps alleviate pain but also enhances your overall well-being. Listening to your body and being mindful of how it responds to different poses will empower you to make informed choices about your routine.

Firstly, it is crucial to assess your current physical condition. Take note of your range of motion, areas of discomfort, and any particular movements that exacerbate your symptoms. Keeping a journal can be beneficial; document how you feel before and after each practice. This information will guide you in selecting poses that suit your needs and help you avoid those that might trigger flare-ups. It is important to be patient with yourself during this assessment phase, as it may take time to understand your body's signals fully.

Once you have a clear understanding of your body's condition, you can begin to select poses that cater to your needs. Focus on gentle, restorative poses that promote flexibility and strength without straining your joints. Poses such as Child's Pose, Cat-Cow Stretch, and Seated Forward Bend are excellent options to start with. Incorporating props, like blocks and straps, can also help modify poses to make them more accessible. The key is to create a balanced routine that includes a mix of restorative poses, gentle stretches, and strengthening exercises, all while ensuring you maintain proper alignment to prevent injury.

In addition to selecting appropriate poses, consider the timing and environment of your practice. Practicing in a calm, quiet space can enhance your experience and help you focus on your movements and breath. You may find that certain times of day work better for you, depending on your energy levels and pain patterns. Morning sessions may invigorate you for the day ahead, while evening practices can help ease tension accumulated throughout the day. Experiment with different times and settings until you find what feels most beneficial for your physical and mental state.

Finally, remember that adapting your routine is an ongoing process. As your body changes and your symptoms fluctuate, your yoga practice should evolve accordingly. Stay open to revisiting and adjusting your poses and routine as needed. Engaging with a knowledgeable instructor who understands arthritis and autoimmune diseases can provide additional support and guidance tailored to your situation. By continuously adapting your routine to meet your current needs, you can cultivate a sustainable yoga practice that not only manages pain but also enhances your quality of life.

Chapter 6: Yoga Sequences for Pain Relief

Morning Routine for Energy and Relief

Establishing a morning routine that fosters energy and relief is crucial for individuals dealing with arthritis and autoimmune diseases. The early hours of the day can set the tone for how one feels both physically and mentally throughout the rest of the day. By incorporating gentle yoga poses, mindfulness practices, and hydration, individuals can create a supportive framework that helps manage pain and increases vitality. This routine emphasizes the importance of listening to one's body and adjusting practices to suit individual needs.

Starting the day with hydration is essential for overall health and can be particularly beneficial for those with arthritis. After a night of rest, the body often wakes up dehydrated, which can exacerbate stiffness and discomfort. Drinking a glass of warm water with a squeeze of lemon can help kickstart the metabolism and promote digestion. This simple act not only hydrates the body but can also provide a refreshing boost that prepares the mind for the day ahead. Following hydration, engaging in deep breathing exercises can enhance oxygen flow and reduce tension, paving the way for a more relaxed state of being.

Incorporating gentle yoga poses into the morning routine can significantly increase flexibility and reduce stiffness. Poses such as Cat-Cow, Child's Pose, and Seated Forward Bend can be performed on a yoga mat or even in bed for those who find it challenging to get up immediately. These poses promote gentle movement, stimulate circulation, and encourage the body to wake up gradually. Each pose should be approached mindfully, focusing on breath and alignment. This awareness not only helps in alleviating physical discomfort but also cultivates a sense of calm and presence, preparing individuals mentally for the day.

Mindfulness and meditation practices are also integral to a morning routine aimed at energy and relief. Taking a few moments to practice mindfulness can enhance emotional well-being and help manage stress, which is often linked to increased pain levels. Simple techniques such as guided imagery or body scans can be effective in promoting relaxation and grounding oneself in the present moment. Setting a positive intention for the day can also be a powerful tool, allowing individuals to cultivate a mindset focused on resilience and self-compassion.

Finally, nourishing the body with a balanced breakfast is key to sustaining energy levels throughout the day. Including anti-inflammatory foods, such as oatmeal topped with berries or a smoothie packed with leafy greens and healthy fats, can provide the necessary nutrients while also supporting joint health. This meal should be enjoyed mindfully, allowing time to savor each bite and appreciate the nourishment being provided. By integrating hydration, gentle movement, mindfulness, and nutritious food into the morning routine, individuals with arthritis and autoimmune diseases can cultivate a sense of energy and relief that empowers them to face daily challenges.

Midday Break for Tension Release

Incorporating a midday break into your routine can serve as an effective strategy for tension release, especially for those living with arthritis or autoimmune diseases. The midday break is not merely a pause from work or daily activities; it is an essential opportunity to reconnect with your body and mind. During this time, gentle yoga practices can alleviate stiffness, reduce pain, and promote a sense of calm. By focusing on mindful breathing and restorative poses, you can create a sanctuary of relief that allows your body to recharge.

One of the primary benefits of a midday break is the reduction of accumulated tension. As the day progresses, it's common to feel the effects of stress and physical strain. For individuals with arthritis, this tension can manifest as heightened pain or discomfort. Engaging in simple yoga stretches during your break can counteract this buildup. Poses such as Cat-Cow, Child's Pose, and Seated Forward Bend can help release tightness in the back, shoulders, and hips, areas often affected by prolonged sitting or repetitive motions.

Breathing exercises are another integral part of a midday tension release routine. Deep, intentional breathing helps oxygenate the body and can lead to a decrease in stress levels. Techniques such as diaphragmatic breathing or the 4-7-8 method can be particularly beneficial. These practices not only enhance relaxation but also improve overall lung capacity and respiratory function, which may be compromised in individuals dealing with chronic conditions. By focusing on your breath, you create a moment of mindfulness that can shift your mental state and provide a respite from daily challenges.

Incorporating restorative poses into your midday break can further enhance the benefits of your practice. Poses like Legs-Up-the-Wall or Supported Bridge Pose allow for gentle stretching while promoting circulation and reducing inflammation. These positions are particularly advantageous for those with arthritis, as they require minimal strain on the joints while still encouraging movement and flexibility. Taking just a few minutes in these restorative poses can significantly improve your overall sense of well-being and ease discomfort.

Finally, creating a dedicated space for your midday break can enhance the effectiveness of your tension release practice. Whether it's a quiet corner of your home or a peaceful spot in a nearby park, having a designated area can signal to your body that it's time to unwind and recharge. Consider incorporating elements that promote relaxation, such as soft music, calming scents, or comfortable props like cushions or blankets. By establishing a routine that prioritizes this midday break, you can cultivate an ongoing practice that not only alleviates pain but also fosters a deeper connection to your body and mind.

Evening Wind-Down for Relaxation

Evening wind-down routines are essential for individuals managing arthritis and autoimmune diseases, as they promote relaxation and prepare the body for restorative sleep. Incorporating gentle yoga poses into your evening routine can significantly alleviate tension and discomfort accumulated throughout the day. These practices not only help in relieving muscle stiffness but also encourage mindfulness, which can be particularly beneficial for those dealing with chronic pain conditions.

Begin your evening wind-down with a few minutes of deep breathing. Find a comfortable seated position, either on the floor or a chair, and close your eyes. Inhale deeply through your nose, allowing your abdomen to expand, and then exhale slowly through your mouth. Focus on your breath, letting go of the stresses and physical discomforts of the day. This mindful breathing can help reduce anxiety and create a sense of calm that is conducive to relaxation.

After establishing a steady breath, transition into gentle stretches that target areas commonly affected by arthritis. The seated forward bend is an excellent choice, as it stretches the spine and hamstrings while promoting relaxation. Sit with your legs extended in front of you, and slowly hinge at the hips, reaching towards your feet. If you can't reach your toes, that's perfectly fine; simply extend your arms as far as you comfortably can. This pose encourages the release of tension in the back and legs, providing a soothing effect on the entire body.

Another beneficial pose is the supported child's pose. This restorative position can help release tension in the hips, back, and shoulders. Kneel on the floor and bring your big toes together, allowing your knees to spread wide. As you lower your torso between your thighs, use a cushion or blanket for support. Rest your forehead on the prop and breathe deeply. This pose not only offers physical relief but also creates a sense of safety and comfort, making it easier to unwind and let go of the day's stresses.

Conclude your evening routine with a few minutes of meditation or mindfulness practice. Simply lying down in a comfortable position, you can focus on your breath or visualize a peaceful scene. This final stage of your wind-down is crucial for signaling to your body that it is time to rest. By incorporating these calming practices into your evening routine, you create a holistic approach to managing pain and enhancing overall well-being, setting the stage for a more restful night and a better day ahead.

Short Sequences for Quick Relief

Short sequences for quick relief can serve as effective tools for individuals managing arthritis and autoimmune diseases. These sequences are designed to be simple yet impactful, enabling practitioners to find immediate comfort and ease in their bodies. The beauty of these sequences lies in their accessibility; they can be performed at home, in a quiet space, or even at the office, allowing for flexibility in practice. By integrating these short routines into daily life, individuals can better manage their symptoms and enhance their overall well-being.

The first sequence focuses on gentle movements to promote circulation and reduce stiffness. It begins with seated cat-cow stretches, allowing for gentle spinal mobilization. Transitioning into neck rolls and shoulder shrugs helps release tension that often accumulates due to prolonged sitting or poor posture. These movements serve to awaken the body and prepare it for further engagement. Practicing this sequence for just five to ten minutes can cultivate a sense of relief and rejuvenation.

Another effective sequence incorporates breath awareness with gentle poses to foster relaxation. Starting with a simple seated forward bend, practitioners can focus on deepening their breath, which is crucial in managing pain and promoting a sense of calm. Following this, a supported child's pose provides a restorative element, allowing the body to surrender and release tension. This sequence emphasizes the connection between breath and movement, creating a holistic approach to relief that can be practiced anytime during the day.

For those seeking to alleviate joint pain specifically, a sequence that targets the major joints can be invaluable. Incorporating movements like ankle rolls, wrist stretches, and gentle hip openers ensures that the body receives attention where it needs it most. Each movement should be executed mindfully, focusing on the range of motion within a comfortable limit. This intentional practice not only enhances joint flexibility but also fosters a deeper awareness of one's body, aiding in the prevention of further discomfort.

Lastly, a restorative sequence can be particularly beneficial for winding down at the end of a day. Poses such as legs-up-the-wall and reclined bound angle can promote relaxation and encourage lymphatic drainage. These soothing poses allow the body to recuperate while providing a sense of grounding. By integrating these restorative practices into a daily routine, individuals can cultivate a sanctuary of relief amidst the challenges posed by arthritis and autoimmune conditions, ultimately enhancing their quality of life.

Chapter 7: Mindfulness and Meditation Techniques

Understanding Mindfulness in Yoga

Mindfulness in yoga is a practice that intertwines awareness and presence with movement and breath. For individuals dealing with arthritis and autoimmune diseases, this approach can be particularly beneficial. Mindfulness involves paying attention to the present moment without judgment, allowing practitioners to cultivate a deeper connection with their bodies. This awareness can help individuals recognize the sensations associated with pain and discomfort, fostering a more compassionate relationship with their physical experiences.

In the context of yoga, mindfulness encourages practitioners to focus on their breath as they move through various poses. This conscious breathing not only aids in relaxation but also serves as an anchor to the present moment. For those managing chronic pain, being mindful of how the body feels during each pose can facilitate adjustments that make the practice more accessible. By tuning into their bodies, individuals can avoid pushing beyond their limits, which is crucial for maintaining a safe and effective yoga routine.

The integration of mindfulness into yoga can also help reduce stress and anxiety, which are common in people with chronic conditions. Stress often exacerbates physical symptoms, leading to a cycle of pain and tension. Mindfulness practices, such as guided meditations or body scans, can enhance emotional well-being by promoting a sense of calm and balance. This mental clarity allows practitioners to approach their physical limitations with a more positive mindset, enabling them to engage with their yoga practice more fully.

Furthermore, mindfulness cultivates a sense of community and support among practitioners. Group classes often emphasize shared experiences, encouraging individuals to connect with others facing similar challenges. This shared mindfulness can foster empathy and understanding, creating an environment where individuals feel safe to explore their practice without fear of judgment. The sense of belonging can be empowering, reinforcing the idea that they are not alone in their journey with arthritis or autoimmune diseases.

Incorporating mindfulness into yoga practice is not just about physical benefits; it also nurtures emotional resilience. Individuals can learn to observe their thoughts and feelings with curiosity rather than reactivity, which can be transformative in managing the psychological aspects of chronic illness. By embracing mindfulness in yoga, those with arthritis and autoimmune diseases can develop a holistic approach to their health, promoting both physical relief and emotional well-being.

Guided Meditations for Pain Management

Guided meditations can be an invaluable tool for individuals coping with arthritis and autoimmune diseases, providing a means to manage pain and enhance overall well-being. These meditative practices focus on cultivating mindfulness and relaxation, which can help individuals shift their attention away from discomfort and foster a sense of peace. By integrating guided meditations into a daily routine, those suffering from chronic pain can develop greater resilience and improve their quality of life.

One common approach in guided meditations for pain management is body scanning. This technique encourages practitioners to mentally scan their bodies from head to toe, observing sensations without judgment. By gently bringing awareness to areas of tension or pain, individuals can learn to acknowledge these feelings without becoming overwhelmed. This process can decrease anxiety and promote relaxation, allowing for a deeper connection between the mind and body, which is crucial for managing the physical manifestations of arthritis.

Another effective method is visualization, where individuals are guided to imagine a peaceful and healing environment. This could be a serene beach, a tranquil forest, or any setting that brings comfort. By immersing themselves in these mental images, practitioners can evoke feelings of safety and calm. Visualization can also involve picturing the body in a state of health and wellness, reinforcing positive thoughts that counteract the negativity often associated with chronic pain. This practice can lead to reduced perceptions of pain and enhanced emotional well-being.

Breath awareness is another key component of guided meditations aimed at pain relief. By focusing on slow, deep breathing, individuals can activate the body's relaxation response. This practice not only reduces stress but also helps in managing pain by promoting the release of endorphins, the body's natural painkillers. Guided meditations that emphasize breath control encourage practitioners to tune into their breath as a tool for calming the mind and body, fostering a sense of empowerment over their pain experience.

Incorporating guided meditations into a holistic approach to managing arthritis and autoimmune diseases can enhance the effectiveness of other therapies, including yoga. The synergy between meditation and physical practice allows for a comprehensive strategy that addresses both mental and physical aspects of pain. As individuals become more adept at using these techniques, they may find increased ease in their yoga practice, leading to improved flexibility, strength, and overall health. By embracing the power of guided meditations, those affected by these chronic conditions can cultivate a more mindful and resilient approach to their pain management journey.

Breathing Techniques for Stress Relief

Breathing techniques play a crucial role in managing stress, especially for individuals dealing with arthritis and autoimmune diseases. Stress can exacerbate pain and inflammation, making it essential to incorporate effective breathing exercises into your daily routine. These techniques not only promote relaxation but also enhance the mind-body connection, fostering a greater sense of calm and well-being. By focusing on breath, individuals can create a natural antidote to the stressors that often accompany chronic pain conditions.

One effective technique is diaphragmatic breathing, which involves engaging the diaphragm fully while inhaling deeply through the nose. This method encourages a more profound intake of oxygen, which is vital for calming the nervous system. To practice, find a comfortable seated or lying position and place one hand on your chest and the other on your abdomen. As you breathe in, ensure that your abdomen rises while your chest remains relatively still. This practice not only helps in reducing anxiety but also improves lung capacity, which can be beneficial for overall health.

Another useful technique is the 4-7-8 breathing pattern, which can be particularly effective in moments of acute stress. Inhale through the nose for a count of four, hold the breath for seven counts, and then exhale through the mouth for a count of eight. This structured approach helps to slow down the heart rate and promote relaxation. Practicing this technique for a few minutes can create a profound sense of tranquility and help alleviate the emotional strain that often accompanies chronic health conditions.

Incorporating mindful breathing into your yoga practice can further enhance its benefits. As you move through various poses, being conscious of your breath allows you to maintain focus and promote relaxation in each posture. For instance, coordinating your inhalations and exhalations with movements can help cultivate a meditative state, distracting the mind from pain and discomfort. This synergy between breath and movement not only enriches the practice but also fosters resilience against the stressors of living with arthritis.

Lastly, regular practice of these breathing techniques can lead to long-term benefits. Over time, individuals may find that they are better equipped to handle stress and pain, resulting in an enhanced quality of life. By dedicating a few minutes each day to focused breathing, those living with arthritis and autoimmune diseases can empower themselves to take control of their emotional and physical well-being. Integrating these practices into your routine can be a simple yet powerful way to cultivate resilience and promote overall health.

Integrating Mindfulness into Daily Life

Integrating mindfulness into daily life can significantly enhance the well-being of individuals living with arthritis and other autoimmune diseases. Mindfulness involves being present in the moment and observing thoughts and sensations without judgment. For those suffering from chronic pain, adopting a mindful approach can help in managing symptoms and reducing stress. By cultivating awareness through mindfulness practices, individuals can learn to recognize pain as a transient experience rather than a constant state, which can alter their relationship with discomfort.

One effective way to incorporate mindfulness is through breath awareness. Practicing deep, intentional breathing can ground individuals in the present moment and provide a calming effect. This technique can be particularly beneficial during moments of heightened pain or anxiety. By focusing on the rhythm of their breath, individuals can create a sense of control over their pain and reduce feelings of helplessness. Establishing a regular breathing practice, such as diaphragmatic breathing or the 4-7-8 technique, can support emotional regulation and promote relaxation throughout the day.

Mindfulness can also be seamlessly integrated into daily activities, transforming mundane tasks into opportunities for presence and awareness. Simple actions, such as washing dishes or walking, can become forms of mindfulness practice. By paying close attention to the sensations involved—such as the warmth of water, the texture of objects, or the rhythm of steps—individuals can foster a deeper connection to their bodies and surroundings. This practice not only enhances the enjoyment of everyday tasks but also cultivates a sense of gratitude for the ability to engage in them, which is particularly significant for those with physical limitations.

Yoga serves as a powerful vehicle for integrating mindfulness into daily life. The combination of mindful movement with breath awareness allows individuals to explore their physical boundaries while remaining present and engaged. Gentle yoga poses can be practiced with an emphasis on mindfulness, encouraging participants to tune into their bodies and notice sensations without judgment. This approach not only helps in managing pain but also fosters a holistic understanding of one's body, leading to increased self-acceptance and reduced anxiety related to chronic conditions.

Lastly, creating a dedicated space and time for mindfulness practice can enhance its integration into daily routines. Setting aside a few minutes each day for mindfulness meditation or yoga can establish a sense of routine and commitment to self-care. This practice can be further supported by journaling reflections on the experience, which can deepen insights and reinforce the benefits of mindfulness. Over time, these small, consistent efforts can lead to profound changes in how individuals with arthritis and autoimmune diseases perceive and manage their pain, ultimately contributing to a more balanced and fulfilling life.

Chapter 8: Overcoming Challenges in Your Practice

Common Obstacles Faced by Practitioners

Practitioners of yoga who are managing arthritis or autoimmune diseases often encounter specific obstacles that can hinder their practice and overall well-being. One of the most common challenges is physical discomfort. Individuals may experience varying degrees of pain and stiffness in their joints, which can make certain poses difficult to perform. This discomfort can lead to frustration and a reluctance to engage fully in the practice. It is essential for practitioners to recognize that modifying poses and listening to their bodies is key to finding a balance between challenge and comfort.

Another significant obstacle is the fear of injury. Many individuals with arthritis or autoimmune diseases may have heightened sensitivity to physical activity due to previous experiences with pain or injury. This fear can create a mental barrier that prevents practitioners from fully exploring their capabilities in yoga. To address this concern, it is crucial for practitioners to work with knowledgeable instructors who can provide guidance on safe modifications and encourage a gentle approach that prioritizes self-care over pushing physical limits.

Motivation can also be a hurdle for practitioners dealing with chronic conditions. The unpredictable nature of arthritis and autoimmune diseases can lead to fluctuations in energy levels and mood, making it challenging to maintain a consistent yoga practice. Practitioners may find that some days are better than others, leading to feelings of discouragement. Establishing a supportive environment, whether through group classes, online communities, or personal affirmations, can help cultivate resilience and foster a sense of accountability that encourages ongoing participation.

Additionally, accessibility to suitable classes and resources can pose a challenge for many practitioners. Not all yoga studios or classes are equipped to accommodate individuals with physical limitations or specific health conditions. This lack of accessibility can discourage those who are interested in yoga from pursuing it further. Practitioners should seek out specialized classes or instructors trained in adaptive yoga practices, ensuring that they receive the support necessary to navigate their unique needs.

Lastly, the integration of mindfulness and mental health practices into yoga can be a complex journey for many practitioners. Chronic pain and the emotional toll of living with a long-term condition can lead to feelings of frustration, anxiety, or depression. Incorporating mindfulness techniques, such as breathwork and meditation, into the practice can enhance the overall experience and provide tools for managing the emotional aspects of their conditions. By acknowledging these obstacles and actively seeking solutions, practitioners can create a more fulfilling and beneficial yoga practice that supports their journey toward pain relief and improved quality of life.

Modifying Poses for Comfort

Modifying poses for comfort is essential for individuals with arthritis and autoimmune diseases, as traditional yoga poses may not always be suitable. Understanding the need for modifications allows practitioners to engage in a safe and effective practice that accommodates their unique physical limitations. By making adjustments, individuals can still experience the benefits of yoga without exacerbating their pain or discomfort. This subchapter will explore various strategies for modifying poses to enhance comfort and accessibility.

One of the primary modifications involves using props such as blocks, straps, and bolsters. These tools can provide additional support and stability, allowing practitioners to maintain proper alignment while reducing strain on the joints. For instance, when performing a seated forward bend, a bolster can be placed on the thighs to allow for a gentler stretch without forcing the body beyond its natural limits. Additionally, blocks can be used to elevate the ground, making it easier to reach the floor without compromising the integrity of the pose.

Another effective approach to modifying poses is to adjust the range of motion. Individuals with arthritis may find that their joints have limited mobility, making it challenging to achieve full expression of a pose. In such cases, it is beneficial to focus on smaller, more comfortable movements. For example, in a gentle twist, instead of aiming for a deep rotation, one can simply turn the torso a few degrees to the side, prioritizing comfort over depth. This allows for the benefits of the pose, such as improved circulation and flexibility, without undue stress on the joints.

The use of supportive seating can also enhance comfort during practice. Practitioners with arthritis may experience difficulty sitting on the floor for extended periods. Utilizing a chair or a yoga bolster can provide a more comfortable option. Adapting poses to a seated position can often reduce strain on the knees and hips. For instance, in a seated mountain pose, one can sit in a chair with feet flat on the ground, focusing on grounding the body and creating a sense of stability while engaging the core.

Finally, listening to the body and honoring its limits is crucial when modifying poses. Every individual's experience with arthritis is unique, and what works for one person may not work for another. Practitioners should be encouraged to explore their own range of comfort and to make adjustments as necessary. This might mean skipping a pose altogether or substituting it with a more accessible variation. Emphasizing the importance of self-awareness and intuition in the practice empowers individuals to take control of their yoga experience, leading to greater enjoyment and long-term adherence to their practice.

Staying Motivated and Consistent

Staying motivated and consistent in a yoga practice is crucial for individuals dealing with arthritis and autoimmune diseases. The benefits of yoga extend beyond physical relief; they also encompass emotional and mental well-being. However, maintaining a regular practice can be challenging, particularly for those experiencing pain or fatigue. Establishing a routine can help cultivate a sense of normalcy and control, which is vital for managing the symptoms associated with these conditions.

One effective strategy for staying motivated is to set realistic and achievable goals. Instead of aiming for perfection, focus on small, incremental improvements. For example, committing to practice yoga for just ten minutes each day can create a sense of accomplishment and encourage progression over time. It can be helpful to track your progress in a journal, noting how you feel before and after each session. Celebrating these small victories can reinforce your commitment and inspire you to continue.

Incorporating variety into your practice can also help maintain motivation. Exploring different yoga styles or poses can prevent boredom and keep you engaged. For those with arthritis, gentle styles such as restorative or chair yoga can be particularly beneficial. Experimenting with various breathing techniques or meditation practices can further enhance your experience and provide additional tools for managing pain. The key is to find what resonates with you and to adapt your routine as needed to suit your current physical and emotional state.

Connecting with a supportive community can significantly enhance motivation and consistency. Joining a local yoga class or an online group can provide encouragement and accountability. Sharing experiences with others who understand the challenges of living with arthritis or autoimmune diseases can foster a sense of belonging. Furthermore, engaging with instructors who specialize in working with individuals with similar conditions can ensure that your practice remains safe and effective.

Lastly, cultivating a positive mindset is essential for long-term commitment to your yoga practice. Recognizing that progress may be slow and that setbacks are a normal part of the journey can help alleviate frustration. Practicing self-compassion and allowing yourself to adjust your goals based on your body's needs are vital. Embracing the journey, regardless of the outcomes, can lead to a deeper appreciation for the practice and its benefits, ultimately leading to greater consistency and motivation in managing arthritis and autoimmune diseases through yoga.

Seeking Support from the Yoga Community

The yoga community offers a wealth of resources for individuals living with arthritis and autoimmune diseases, providing not only physical support but also emotional and social connections. Engaging with this community can enhance one's yoga practice and overall well-being. Local studios often host classes specifically designed for individuals with chronic pain and mobility issues, allowing participants to experience yoga in a supportive environment. These classes are typically led by instructors trained in adaptive techniques, ensuring that modifications are available to accommodate various levels of ability.

Online platforms further expand access to the yoga community, creating a space where individuals can connect regardless of geographical limitations. Virtual classes, workshops, and forums enable people to share their experiences and seek guidance from others who understand the challenges posed by arthritis and autoimmune conditions. These online resources can be particularly beneficial for those who may find it difficult to attend in-person classes due to pain or fatigue. Furthermore, many reputable yoga instructors and therapists share valuable insights through webinars and social media, fostering a sense of belonging and shared purpose.

Support groups within the yoga community can provide a unique avenue for connection. These groups often meet regularly to practice yoga together while also offering a platform for participants to discuss their struggles and triumphs. This exchange of experiences can be incredibly empowering, reminding individuals that they are not alone in their journey. Establishing relationships with fellow practitioners can lead to increased motivation and encouragement, reinforcing the commitment to a regular yoga practice that can alleviate symptoms associated with arthritis and autoimmune diseases.

In addition to group classes and support networks, many yoga communities emphasize the importance of workshops that focus on specialized techniques for managing pain and stress. These workshops often address the emotional aspects of living with chronic illness and teach participants how to integrate mindfulness and breathwork into their daily lives. By learning these skills in a community setting, individuals can gain practical tools for coping with the ups and downs of their conditions, ultimately enhancing their quality of life.

Finally, seeking support from the yoga community can foster a holistic approach to health that includes not only physical activity but also lifestyle changes and self-care practices. Many yoga practitioners advocate for a balanced diet, meditation, and other wellness strategies that complement a consistent yoga practice. By engaging with the community, individuals can explore these additional avenues for support, leading to a more comprehensive understanding of how to manage their arthritis or autoimmune disease. This collective knowledge can empower individuals to take charge of their health, transforming their yoga journey into a vital part of their healing process.

Chapter 9: Testimonials and Success Stories

Real-Life Experiences from Practitioners

Practitioners of yoga who live with arthritis and autoimmune diseases often share transformative experiences that highlight the profound impact of this practice on their lives. Many report a significant reduction in pain levels and improved mobility as they incorporate gentle yoga poses into their daily routines. Through personal stories, these individuals reveal how yoga has not only alleviated physical discomfort but has also fostered a sense of emotional well-being. Their journeys exemplify the therapeutic potential of yoga as a complementary approach to managing chronic conditions.

One practitioner, diagnosed with rheumatoid arthritis, discovered yoga after struggling with limitations in her daily activities. Initially hesitant, she attended a gentle yoga class tailored for individuals with chronic pain. Over time, she learned to listen to her body and modify poses to suit her needs. Through consistent practice, she found that her joints felt less stiff and her range of motion improved. This positive change encouraged her to become more active overall, embracing a lifestyle that included walking and even hiking, activities she had once thought were behind her.

Another remarkable story comes from a man living with ankylosing spondylitis, a form of arthritis that can lead to significant back pain and stiffness. He began practicing yoga as part of a holistic approach to his condition, combining it with physical therapy and medication. His experience with specific poses designed to enhance spinal flexibility made a noticeable difference. He found that yoga not only provided physical relief but also helped him manage stress and anxiety associated with his illness. This dual benefit of physical and mental wellness has been a recurring theme among many practitioners.

In addition to physical benefits, participants in yoga classes report a shift in their mindset toward their conditions. One woman, diagnosed with lupus, emphasized the importance of community and support found in her yoga class. The shared experiences and understanding among fellow practitioners created a safe space where she felt empowered to confront her challenges. The camaraderie fostered through yoga practice enabled her to build resilience and develop coping strategies, ultimately enhancing her quality of life despite her diagnosis.

These real-life experiences underscore the importance of a tailored approach to yoga for those with arthritis and autoimmune diseases. Each practitioner's journey highlights the adaptability of yoga, allowing individuals to find their own path to healing. As they share their stories, they inspire others facing similar challenges to explore yoga as a viable, beneficial practice. The collective wisdom of these practitioners serves as a testament to the potential of yoga to improve not only physical health but also emotional and social well-being for those living with chronic conditions.

The Impact of Yoga on Daily Life

The integration of yoga into daily life can significantly enhance the well-being of individuals living with arthritis and autoimmune diseases. Yoga is more than just a physical practice; it encompasses mindfulness, breathing techniques, and meditative elements that contribute to overall health. For those managing chronic pain, the gentle movements and stretches of yoga can promote increased flexibility and strength. This can lead to improved mobility, enabling individuals to engage more fully in daily activities, which is crucial for maintaining independence.

One of the most profound impacts of yoga is its ability to reduce stress and anxiety, conditions that often accompany chronic illnesses. The practice encourages a focus on breath, which can activate the body's relaxation response and lower cortisol levels. This reduction in stress can lead to decreased inflammation in the body, a significant benefit for those with arthritis and autoimmune disorders. By fostering a sense of calm and mindfulness, yoga provides a valuable tool for managing the emotional challenges of living with chronic pain.

Additionally, yoga promotes better sleep patterns, which are often disrupted in individuals with arthritis and autoimmune diseases. The calming effects of yoga can help establish a more consistent bedtime routine and improve the quality of sleep. Better rest is essential for recovery and managing pain, as inadequate sleep can exacerbate symptoms and lead to a cycle of discomfort. Incorporating restorative yoga poses into the evening can signal to the body that it is time to wind down, further promoting relaxation and restorative sleep.

Yoga also fosters community and support, which can be particularly beneficial for those facing the challenges of chronic illness. Many yoga studios offer classes specifically designed for individuals with arthritis and other autoimmune conditions, creating a safe space where participants can share their experiences and support one another. This sense of belonging can mitigate feelings of isolation and empower individuals to take an active role in their health. The shared experience of practicing yoga together can enhance motivation and accountability, making it easier to maintain a consistent practice.

In conclusion, the impact of yoga on daily life for individuals with arthritis and autoimmune diseases is multifaceted. By incorporating yoga into their routines, individuals can experience improvements in flexibility, strength, stress management, sleep quality, and social support. These benefits collectively contribute to a greater sense of control over their health and well-being. As a gentle and adaptable practice, yoga can be tailored to meet the unique needs of each individual, making it an invaluable resource in the journey toward pain relief and enhanced quality of life.

Lessons Learned from the Journey

The journey of incorporating yoga into the lives of those with arthritis and autoimmune diseases has revealed valuable lessons that extend beyond the physical practice itself. One of the most significant insights is the importance of listening to one's body. Individuals often push through discomfort, seeking to achieve specific poses or routines. However, learning to recognize and respect the body's signals is crucial. This awareness fosters a more sustainable practice, allowing individuals to adapt their movements according to their daily fluctuations in pain and energy levels.

Another important lesson is the power of consistency. Establishing a regular yoga practice can be challenging, especially on days when symptoms flare up. Yet, those who commit to a consistent routine often experience cumulative benefits over time. This consistency not only helps improve flexibility and strength but also cultivates a sense of routine and stability in a life that can often feel unpredictable due to chronic conditions. The act of showing up for oneself, regardless of the intensity of the practice, is a testament to resilience.

Community support is another key takeaway from this journey. Engaging with others who share similar struggles can provide emotional and motivational benefits that enhance the yoga experience. Whether through local classes or online forums, sharing stories and tips can create a sense of belonging and understanding. This connection is particularly important for those dealing with chronic pain, as it reinforces the notion that they are not alone in their experiences and challenges.

Mindfulness, cultivated through yoga, has also emerged as a profound lesson. Practicing mindfulness encourages individuals to remain present and engaged with their feelings, both physical and emotional. This awareness can lead to a deeper understanding of how stress and anxiety can exacerbate pain, prompting individuals to develop coping strategies that integrate mindfulness into daily life. By focusing on breath and movement, practitioners learn to find calm amidst the chaos of chronic illness.

Finally, the journey has underscored the importance of patience. Progress in yoga and life with arthritis is often non-linear, marked by ups and downs. Embracing patience allows individuals to celebrate small victories, whether it's achieving a new pose or simply feeling more comfortable in their skin. Recognizing that improvement takes time can help mitigate frustration and foster a more compassionate relationship with oneself. Through these lessons, practitioners can cultivate a more enriching and empowering yoga experience tailored to their unique needs.

Inspiring Others to Begin Their Practice

Inspiring others to begin their yoga practice, especially those living with arthritis and autoimmune diseases, is a vital step toward fostering a supportive community. Many individuals in these circumstances may feel overwhelmed by their condition, leading to hesitation about starting any form of physical activity. However, sharing personal stories of transformation and the benefits of yoga can motivate them to embark on their journey. Emphasizing the gentle and adaptable nature of yoga allows potential practitioners to see that it is not only accessible but can be tailored to their unique needs.

One effective approach is to highlight the physical benefits of yoga for those with arthritis and autoimmune diseases. Research has shown that regular yoga practice can improve flexibility, reduce pain, and enhance overall mobility. Demonstrating how specific poses can alleviate common symptoms associated with these conditions can create a sense of hope. When individuals understand that yoga can be a tool for pain management and improved function, they may be more inclined to give it a try.

Additionally, it is essential to emphasize the mental and emotional benefits of yoga. Living with chronic pain can lead to feelings of isolation, frustration, and anxiety. Yoga offers a sanctuary where individuals can cultivate mindfulness and develop coping strategies. By sharing techniques such as breathwork and meditation, practitioners can inspire others to view yoga as a holistic approach to wellness that addresses both body and mind. This dual benefit can be a compelling reason for individuals to start their practice.

Community plays a significant role in encouraging individuals to begin their yoga journey. Creating a supportive environment where those with arthritis and autoimmune diseases can practice together fosters camaraderie and understanding. Group classes designed specifically for these conditions can provide a safe space for individuals to share their experiences and challenges. Highlighting success stories from fellow practitioners can create a sense of belonging and motivate others to participate, knowing they are not alone in their struggles.

Finally, offering resources and guidance can further inspire others to start their practice. Providing information on accessible classes, online tutorials, and instructional materials can eliminate barriers to entry. Encouraging individuals to start their practice at home, even with just a few simple poses, can ease them into the routine. By empowering them with knowledge and support, they are more likely to feel confident in their ability to begin and maintain a yoga practice that enhances their quality of life despite the challenges they face.

Chapter 10: Resources and Further Reading

Recommended Books and Guides

In navigating the journey of managing arthritis and autoimmune diseases, integrating yoga into daily routines can be significantly beneficial. To support this endeavor, there are several recommended books and guides that provide valuable insights, pose instructions, and mindful practices tailored specifically for individuals with these conditions. These resources can enhance one's understanding of the therapeutic aspects of yoga while offering practical tools for alleviating pain and improving overall quality of life.

One essential resource is "Yoga for Arthritis" by Ellen Saltonstall and Dr. Steffany Moonaz. This book combines the expertise of a seasoned yoga instructor and a medical professional, providing a comprehensive approach to using yoga as a therapeutic tool for arthritis. It includes detailed descriptions of poses, modifications, and sequences that cater to varying levels of mobility. The authors emphasize the importance of listening to one's body, making this guide particularly valuable for those dealing with the fluctuating symptoms of arthritis and autoimmune diseases.

Another noteworthy title is "The Yoga of Healing" by B.K.S. Iyengar. Though not solely focused on arthritis, Iyengar's work is foundational in the world of yoga therapy. His emphasis on alignment and the use of props allows individuals with limited mobility to practice safely. This book offers a variety of poses and sequences that can be adapted for those experiencing chronic pain, and its holistic approach encourages practitioners to cultivate a deeper connection between the mind and body, which is vital for managing chronic conditions.

For those seeking a more guided experience, "The Complete Guide to Yin Yoga" by Bernie Clark provides an excellent resource. Yin yoga is a slower-paced style that emphasizes long-held postures, which can be particularly therapeutic for joint pain and stiffness. This guide not only explains the physical benefits of yin yoga but also delves into the philosophy behind the practice. It offers insights into how slow, mindful movements can help release tension and promote healing, making it a suitable option for those with arthritis and similar ailments.

Lastly, "Yoga for the Inflexible" by Lollye and Mark R. Miller is a practical guide that addresses the unique challenges faced by individuals with limited flexibility. This book focuses on gentle stretches and movements that can be beneficial for those with autoimmune diseases, emphasizing the importance of patience and gradual progress. With clear instructions and modifications for each pose, it serves as an excellent companion for anyone looking to incorporate yoga into their self-care regimen while managing the symptoms of arthritis. Each of these recommended books and guides offers unique perspectives and tools to empower individuals on their healing journeys through yoga.

Online Resources and Communities

The rise of the internet has transformed the way people seek information and support for conditions like arthritis and autoimmune diseases. Online resources have become invaluable tools for patients looking to manage their symptoms and enhance their well-being through holistic practices like yoga. Websites dedicated to arthritis education provide a wealth of knowledge, including the latest research findings, treatment options, and lifestyle advice. Many of these platforms are run by reputable medical organizations, ensuring that the information is accurate and trustworthy.

In addition to educational websites, numerous online communities offer a space for individuals to connect with others facing similar challenges. Forums and social media groups enable participants to share their experiences, seek advice, and provide encouragement. Engaging with others who understand the realities of living with arthritis or autoimmune diseases can foster a sense of belonging and reduce feelings of isolation. These communities often serve as a source of motivation, where members can discuss their yoga journeys and share tips for incorporating poses into their daily routines.

Many yoga instructors and therapists have recognized the need for accessible resources tailored specifically to those with arthritis and related conditions. Online classes, workshops, and instructional videos are widely available, allowing individuals to practice yoga in the comfort of their own homes. These resources often highlight modifications and gentle approaches to ensure safety and effectiveness, accommodating various levels of flexibility and strength. This flexibility in learning allows individuals to progress at their own pace, making yoga a more approachable and sustainable practice for pain relief.

Moreover, the wealth of online resources extends to blogs and personal stories that can inspire and educate. Many individuals living with arthritis share their personal journeys, detailing how yoga has impacted their lives. These narratives not only provide practical insights into specific poses and routines but also emphasize the emotional benefits of yoga, such as improved mental health and resilience. By reading about others' successes and challenges, individuals can gain a deeper understanding of how to adapt yoga to their unique situations.

Lastly, online resources often feature expert opinions and interviews with healthcare professionals who specialize in arthritis and autoimmune diseases. These insights can help individuals make informed decisions about their yoga practice and overall health management. By accessing expert advice, patients can learn how to integrate yoga into their treatment plans safely. This comprehensive approach ensures that individuals do not feel overwhelmed by their conditions but rather empowered to take control of their health through informed choices and community support.

Finding Qualified Instructors

Finding qualified instructors who can effectively teach yoga to individuals with arthritis and autoimmune diseases is crucial for ensuring a safe and beneficial practice. Not all yoga instructors possess the specialized knowledge required to accommodate the unique needs of this population. When seeking an instructor, it is important to prioritize those with specific training in teaching yoga to individuals with chronic pain or related conditions. Look for certifications from reputable organizations that emphasize adaptive techniques and awareness of physical limitations.

One effective approach to finding the right instructor is to seek recommendations from healthcare professionals, such as rheumatologists or physical therapists, who are familiar with the specific needs of patients with arthritis. These professionals often have a network of reputable yoga instructors who specialize in therapeutic practices. Additionally, local arthritis support groups can be valuable resources, as members may share their experiences and recommend instructors who have successfully taught them.

When evaluating potential instructors, inquire about their experience working with individuals who have arthritis or autoimmune diseases. It is essential that the instructor understands modification techniques for various poses to accommodate different levels of mobility and pain. A qualified instructor should be able to demonstrate an awareness of the symptoms associated with these conditions and create a supportive environment where students feel safe to express their limitations and concerns.

In addition to experience, assess the instructor's approach to teaching. An effective instructor will prioritize communication, ensuring that students feel comfortable discussing their health issues and any pain they may experience during practice. Look for instructors who encourage feedback and adjust their teaching style accordingly, fostering an inclusive and understanding atmosphere. This approach not only enhances the practice but also helps build trust between the instructor and students, which is essential for those managing chronic conditions.

Finally, consider attending a few trial classes to gauge the instructor's teaching style and the class environment. Observe how the instructor interacts with students and whether they provide individualized attention. A good instructor will demonstrate patience, understanding, and a willingness to adapt practices to meet individual needs. By finding a qualified instructor who aligns with these criteria, individuals with arthritis and autoimmune diseases can experience the profound benefits of yoga in a way that is safe and supportive.

Continuing Your Yoga Journey

Continuing your yoga journey after beginning a practice tailored for arthritis and autoimmune diseases involves both commitment and adaptability. As you progress, it is essential to listen to your body and honor its limitations while also encouraging growth. Regular practice can help maintain flexibility, improve strength, and reduce pain, but it's vital to approach your routine with mindfulness and patience. Consistency in your practice will yield the best results, so aim to incorporate yoga into your daily life, even if only for a few minutes each day.

As you deepen your practice, consider exploring various styles of yoga that may suit your needs. Restorative yoga, for instance, focuses on gentle stretches and relaxation, making it ideal for those with chronic pain. Yin yoga, on the other hand, emphasizes longer-held poses that promote joint mobility and deep tissue release. Finding the right style can help you enjoy the benefits of yoga while accommodating your specific condition. Additionally, seeking classes specifically designed for individuals with arthritis can provide a supportive environment and foster a sense of community.

Setting realistic goals is another essential aspect of continuing your yoga journey. Rather than aiming for perfection, focus on gradual improvements. Celebrate small victories, whether it's holding a pose for a few extra breaths or experiencing less discomfort in your joints. Keeping a journal of your progress can help you stay motivated and provide insight into how your body responds to different practices. Remember, yoga is a personal journey, and it's important to honor your unique path.

Incorporating mindfulness and breathing techniques into your practice can enhance your overall experience. Pranayama, or breath control, can help alleviate stress and promote relaxation, which is particularly beneficial for those managing chronic conditions. Mindfulness encourages you to be present in the moment, allowing you to tune into your body's signals and adjust your practice as needed. These tools can empower you to navigate challenges and build resilience on your journey toward better health.

Finally, connecting with others who share similar experiences can provide encouragement and support. Consider joining a local or online yoga community focused on arthritis and autoimmune diseases. Sharing your journey with others can help you feel less isolated and more inspired. Participating in workshops, classes, or retreats can also deepen your understanding of yoga and introduce you to new techniques and philosophies. Your yoga journey is a lifelong process, and engaging with a supportive community can make it more enriching and enjoyable.

Disclaimer:

- **Purpose**: The book is for informational or educational purposes only.
- **Liability**: The author and publisher are not responsible for any loss or adverse effects that may arise from the book's information.
- **Consultation**: Readers should consult their own medical advisors for advice on their condition and treatment.
- **Accuracy**: The author has made every effort to provide accurate information, but the book may contain errors or omissions.
- **Verification**: Readers should verify any information independently.

"The author has made every attempt to provide information that is accurate and complete, but this book is not intended as a substitute for professional medical advice".

My Story

www.yogawithcarol.org

I became a qualified Yoga Instructor because I suffer from Rheumatoid Arthritis. I was diagnosed in 2020 and I am 50 years old. Integrating Yoga into my daily routine had such a positive effect on my day to day life that I trained in Yoga so that I could help others. When I started Yoga I struggled to walk across a room or to pick things up due to the severity of the pain, stiffness and swelling, and I was miserable. I had always been reasonably fit and healthy and found it difficult to accept. **Yoga has transformed my life!** It has increased my mobility, reduced my pain and swelling, given me back my physical fitness so that I can enjoy life and cope with being a single Mother of 2.

I now do Yoga everyday as well as teaching various classes a week both online and in person. I also run a few times a week and have just signed up to run my first marathon in 2025.

If you are suffering, you ache when you are in bed at night, you wake up sore, stiff and swollen in the morning and your mental and physical health are suffering because of it, then I encourage you to try Yoga and see what difference it can make to **YOUR** life.

Come and join us at Yoga with Carol or find a local yoga studio and venture to your first class. Yoga is for **everyone** and can be **adapted** to suit your needs. The difference will **amaze** you.

Namaste

Carol

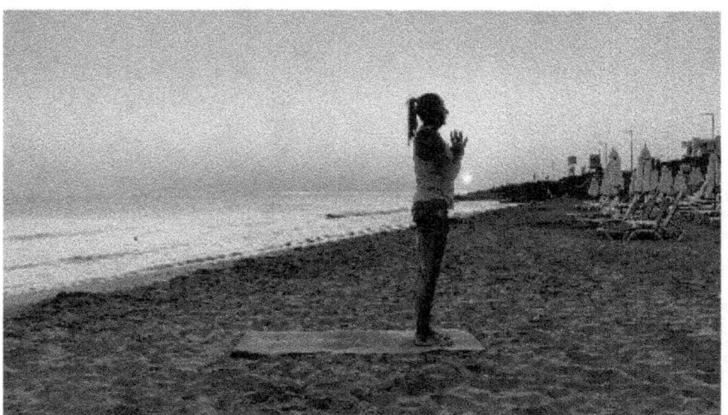

Picture by Carol Findlay

www.ingramcontent.com/pod-product-compliance
Lightning Source LLC
Chambersburg PA
CBHW071044250726
48653CB00005B/2000